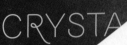

CRYSTAL

A LITTLE INTR...
TO TH...

N

RP | NIS

PHILADELPHIA

RP Minis™
Hachette Book Group
1290 Avenue of the Americas,
New York, NY 10104
www.runningpress.com
@Running_Press

Printed in China

First Edition: September 2020

Published by RP Minis, an imprint of Perseus Books, LLC, a subsidiary of Hachette Book Group, Inc. The RP Minis name and logo is a trademark of the Hachette Book Group.

The Hachette Speakers Bureau provides a wide range of authors for speaking events. To find out more, go to www.hachettespeakersbureau.com or call (866) 376-6591.

Text by Nikki Van De Car | Design by Amanda Richmond

Library of Congress Control Number: 2020931539

ISBN: 978-0-7624-9795-9

LREX

10 9 8 7 6 5

CRYSTALS

A LITTLE INTRODUCTION
TO THEIR POWERS

NIKKI VAN DE CAR

ILLUSTRATIONS BY
ANISA MAKHOUL

RP MINIS

PHILADELPHIA

RP Minis™
Hachette Book Group
1290 Avenue of the Americas,
New York, NY 10104
www.runningpress.com
@Running_Press

Printed in China

First Edition: September 2020

Published by RP Minis, an imprint of Perseus Books, LLC, a subsidiary of Hachette Book Group, Inc. The RP Minis name and logo is a trademark of the Hachette Book Group.

The Hachette Speakers Bureau provides a wide range of authors for speaking events. To find out more, go to www.hachettespeakersbureau.com or call (866) 376-6591.

Text by Nikki Van De Car | Design by Amanda Richmond

Library of Congress Control Number: 2020931539

ISBN: 978-0-7624-9795-9

LREX

10 9 8 7 6 5

CONTENTS

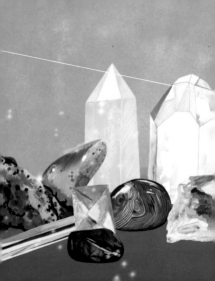

INTRODUCTION

WE OFTEN THINK OF CRYSTALS as rocks that are just really pretty. And there's some truth to that! Crystals are formed when liquid matter cools and hardens in such a way that the molecules sort themselves into a repeating pattern, which is what makes them so lovely and forms them into such interesting shapes.

But there's more to these stones than just aesthetics. Crystals are millions of years old, and they are a way to help us connect with the power of the earth and the very molecules that make up the universe. Those incredibly specific molecular geometric patterns create vibrations that allow crystals to store and harness specific energies and information. Clear quartz, for instance, is used in watches, memory chips, ultrasound devices, and more as a way to store information like an unchanging time or a steady frequency. If electronics can harness this power then so can we, on a more basic, natural level.

In fact, crystals have been used in these ways for thousands of years. Our ancestors incorporated crystals into healing rituals, divination practices, burial rites, 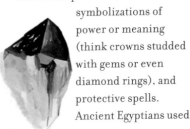 symbolizations of power or meaning (think crowns studded with gems or even diamond rings), and protective spells. Ancient Egyptians used

peridot to ward off nightmares,
and ancient Greeks used
amethyst to prevent intoxication
(or perhaps just the resulting
hangover).

There are several different
shapes of crystals, and each can
be used in a different way.

WAND

Rough at one end and pointed at the other, these kinds of stones are often used in jewelry or as protective amulets. They can also be used to activate crystal grids, as this shape allows you to direct the crystal's energies in a more targeted way.

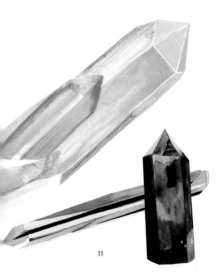

11

CHUNK

The larger crystals you see are often chunk crystals. They have essentially been mined and presented as is, so geodes, uncut turquoise, pyrite, etc. are considered chunk crystals. These larger examples release their energy in a more diffuse way than small or shaped stones, so they're good for general household use.

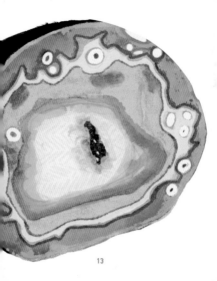

CUT

This is when a crystal or gem has been shaped to enhance sparkle and capture light, which amplifies the crystal's energies, making it even more powerful.

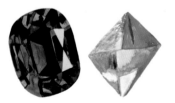

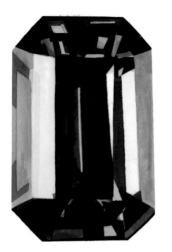

15

TUMBLED

These are the stones you'll find
in bins at a science or mystical
shop. They are smooth, shiny,
and comforting to hold.

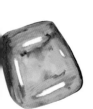

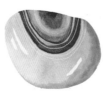

TYPES OF CRYSTALS

THE FIRST STEP IN CHOOSING
a crystal to work with is to deter-
mine your needs at the moment.
Ask yourself questions. Are you
addressing a physical ailment or

a spiritual one? Sometimes you might find yourself drawn to a particular stone, so that the stone chooses you, rather than the other way around. When you are looking to add a new crystal to your collection, start by following your instincts—what attracts you? You should pay attention to aesthetics here, because what seems like an attraction on a purely visual level might be your mind telling you exactly what you need. Then hold the stone in your hand. Does it feel warm or cool? Do you feel any vibrations or pulses? What is your emotional response? If you feel in resonance with the stone, then it is right for you.

It's possible, even likely, that from time to time you will need a combination of stones, such as

obsidian, hematite, and pyrite
for protection, or amethyst and
lapis lazuli for intuition. Trust
your instincts.

And if you're not sure, try
clear quartz. It's the salt in the
spice cabinet of crystals.

Common Stones and Their Uses

AGATE

Invites courage, strength,
and self-confidence.

ALEXANDRITE

A detoxifying crystal that can
help control anxiety and aid in
finding emotional maturity.

AMAZONITE

Protects against
electromagnetic stress
and seasonal affective
disorder. Encourages self-
determination and
leadership abilities.

AMETHYST

Develops intuition and
spiritual awareness.
Aids in meditation,
calm, and tranquility.
Relieves headaches.

APATITE

Brings out the best version
of yourself, and heals
the bones and teeth.

APOPHYLLITE

A calming stone that cleanses
the third eye and crown
chakras, releasing tension.

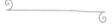

AQUAMARINE

Aids in expressing your
personal truth. Reduces
fear and tension.

AVENTURINE

This "stone of opportunity"
invites luck and wealth.

AZURITE

Helps find spiritual or psychic blocks that are causing physical blocks. Transforms fear into understanding. Good for arthritis and joint pain.

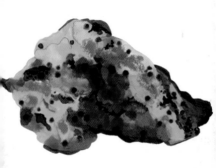

BISMUTH

Aids in self-reflection, and calms and soothes the mind. Can diffuse electromagnetic energies and help organize a chaotic mind.

BLACK
TOURMALINE

A stone of protection.
Places an energetic boundary
between you and the energy
of those around you.

BLOODSTONE

Helps you find your inner strength and tap into your courage and vitality.

BLUE LACE AGATE
This gentle stone of communication helps alleviate anger and tension.

BRONZITE
Energizes and protects, so that you have the strength and backup needed to tackle any challenges.

CALCITE

An energy amplifier,
it eases communication
between the physical
and spiritual world.

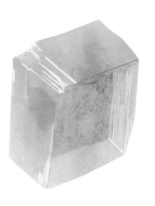

35

CARNELIAN

Enhances creativity and sexuality, and helps with exploring past-life experiences. Aids in digestion and soothes menstrual pain.

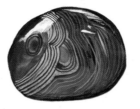

CELESTITE

Allows you to stand back
and look at a problem
without emotional clouding.
Clears any blocks that may
be preventing you from
connecting with
the spirit world.

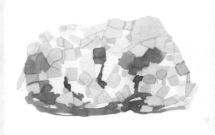

39

CITRINE

A stone of abundance,
it invites success and
money and raises self-esteem.
Good for the heart, kidneys,
liver, and muscles.

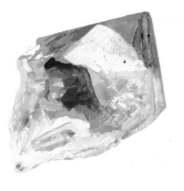

41

CLEAR QUARTZ

A stone of healing, it channels power and amplifies universal energy. This stone can be programmed to whatever use you require.

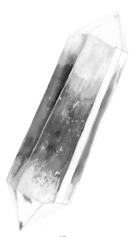

43

DIAMOND

Symbolizes purity and
innocence, and encourages
truth and trust.

EMERALD

The "stone of successful love,"
emerald encourages you to
give and receive love.

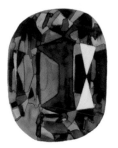

FLUORITE

Useful in decision-making and
helps with concentration.

FUCHSITE

The "healer's stone,"
fuchsite allows you to see
the truth with love.

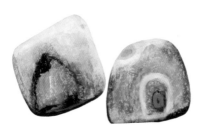

GARNET

A stone of health and creativity, it stimulates your internal fire. Wards off cancer, is good for skin elasticity, and also helps prevent nightmares.

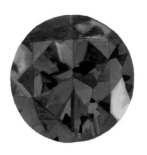

HEMATITE

A stone of protection and grounding, it closes your aura to keep out negative energy. Provides support for astral projection.

HOWLITE

Eliminates anger so that you can approach a situation with a calm heart and a clear mind.

IOLITE

Balances male and
female energies and aids
in self-acceptance.

JADE

Will inspire you to
ambition and keep you
working toward your
objective. Good for
longevity.

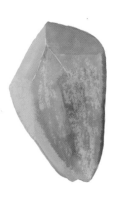

KYANITE

This crystal will help
you align with your spirit
guides, and can alleviate
muscle pain.

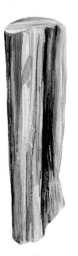

55

LABRADORITE

Helps you see past any
blocks or illusions
to divine your
true life's work.

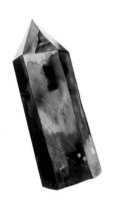

57

LAPIS LAZULI

A stone of focus, it helps amplify thought, aids in meditation and releases from melancholy. Good for sore throats and fever.

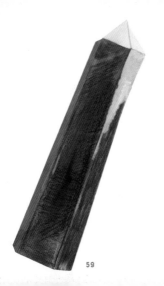

59

LEPIDOLITE
Encourages independence
and self-sufficiency.

MALACHITE
Releases stored emotions, and
allows you to look inward.

MERLINITE

A "stone of storms," merlinite
can help those who have been
hurt move forward in life.

MOOKAITE

A stone of adventure,
mookaite will give you
direction and a sense of
the power of your own
possibilities.

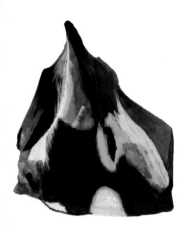

MOONSTONE

Soothes the emotions as
well as the digestive system.
Encourages peace and
harmony within.

MORGANITE

A useful stone for teachers,
morganite helps you to love
without attachment.

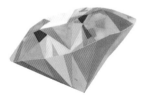

OBSIDIAN

A stone of protection,
particularly from spiritual
forces. It will help you
understand and face your
deepest fears. Helps with
bacterial and viral invasions.

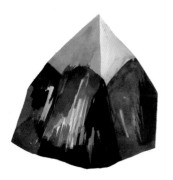

OPAL

Stone of amplification,
it enhances mystical
experiences and creativity.
Balances mood swings.

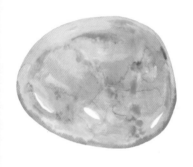

PERIDOT

Used since ancient
times as a symbol of
the sun, it invites energy,
positivity, and light.

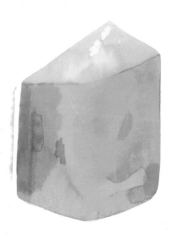

71

PYRITE

Stone of defense
and protection, it
symbolizes the sun and
cleanses the blood.

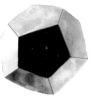

RHODOCHROSITE

A stone of self-love
that helps you recover
from emotional wounds.

RHODONITE

A calming stone that allows
you to accept love.

ROSE QUARTZ

A stone of love, not just romantic love, but familial and brotherly love as well. Nurturing and comforting, this stone dissipates anger.

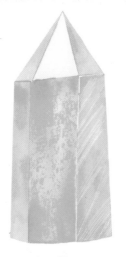

RUBY

The "stone of divine
creativity," ruby inspires
energy, passion,
and power.

RUTILATED QUARTZ

This type of quartz is
threaded with golden veins
known as "angel threads" or
"Venus hairs." It can aid in
combatting depression and
can strengthen your will.

SAPPHIRE

A stone of wisdom that can
ease depression, anxiety, and
insomnia as well as heal eye
and blood disorders.

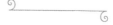

SARDONYX

A stone of courage that can
bring happiness and balance
to romantic relationships.

SELENITE

A form of gypsum crystals
often in wand shape, selenite
is used for clearing and
purifying negative energies,
and activating positive ones.

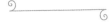

SERPENTINE

Regulates hormones
and allows the body to
come into balance.

SHATTUCKITE

Aids in processing and understanding psychic experiences.

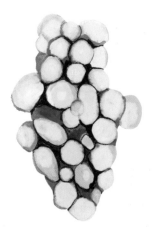

83

SHUNGITE

A detoxifying stone that
can also help shield
you from the effects of
electromagnetic radiation.

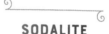

SODALITE

A "stone of truth," sodalite
will help you speak your own
truth, as well as accept the
truths of others, no matter
how hard they may be to hear.

SMOKY QUARTZ

A stone of protection,
it stimulates your survival
instincts. Enhances
focus and fertility.

SUGILITE

Represents perfect spiritual love, and gives a sense of belonging. Can ease pain and mental health issues.

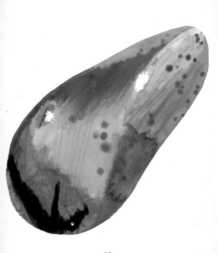

87

SUNSTONE

An antidepressant that
stimulates the kidneys and
allows energy to flow freely
throughout the body.

TIGER'S EYE

A stone of stability, it
enhances personal power
and integrity.

TURQUOISE

A stone of healing, it
guards against disease and
environmental pollutants.

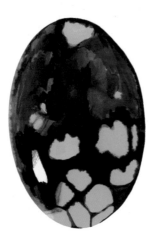

91

YELLOW JASPER

Stimulates the pancreas and the endocrine system, and helps align the energy meridians.

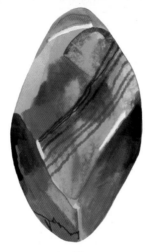

93

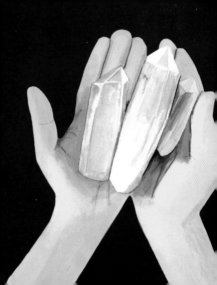

CHOOSING AND ACTIVATING YOUR CRYSTAL

ONCE YOU'VE CHOSEN A STONE,
you'll want to clear it. Your stone

didn't come to you straight from the earth—it was found by others, packaged by others, and handled by others, and their energies have penetrated it. There are several ways to purify your crystal: soaking it in saltwater or holding it under running water (preferably a stream, but rain or even your faucet will do in a pinch) are the simplest ways, but if your stone is a bit too delicate

for that, you can let it rest with
carnelian or clear quartz, which
have cleansing properties. You
can also do a little smudging,
or let sunlight or moonlight
work their magic.

Once the stone is cleared,
it can be activated. While each
stone always carries its special
properties within itself, you
can enhance a stone's power
by programming it with your

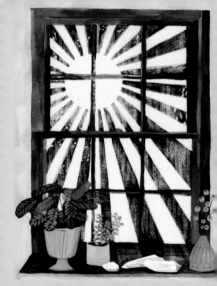

specific needs and intentions. Clear quartz in particular can become whatever you need it to be, and do whatever you need it to do.

Activating your crystal can take any form you want it to. It can be as simple as holding the crystal in your hand and setting an intention. Feel free to invoke a higher power, or you can really set the stage for your healing process by performing a ritual. You can create any kind of ritual you want, but here is an example to get you started.

STAND IN NATURAL LIGHT.

This could be light from a candle, sunlight, or moonlight. Cup the crystal in your palms, allowing the light to fall on it. Now, focus on the crystal with your intention in mind. This can be something very general, like an overall sense of positivity or healing, but you can also get very specific. If you are having difficulty sleeping, for instance, hold a sapphire or moonstone in your palm and imagine a peaceful night's rest. You can speak this intention aloud, or whisper it in your heart. Then, close your palm to seal your intention, bowing your head.

Uses

Because there are so many
stones with such varied uses,
crystal healing can be a fairly
complicated practice. The effect
of each crystal changes not just
with its type but also its shape
and how it has been activated
and cleansed. For instance, rose
quartz will produce different

results depending on whether it is shaped as a wand or left as a tumbled stone, as well as the intentions you gave it during activation.

For generalized use, you can get a large geode and place it in a specific location. For instance, you can keep an amethyst next to your bed to promote sleep, blue lace agate in your dining room to keep the lines of communication clear, or lapis lazuli on your altar to enhance your connection to the spirit world.

It can be helpful to keep smaller, tumbled stones in your pocket or at your place of work to help you throughout the day. If you are having a difficult phone conversation, you can hold aquamarine, howlite, or pyrite in your palm to help keep you calm and centered. If you're

working on a paper or studying,
keep bismuth, fluorite, and jade
handy, and if you're trying for a
new job or spending a weekend
in Vegas, you should definitely
bring aventurine and citrine.

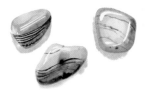

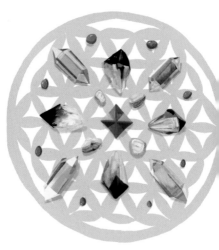

Crystal Grids

While every crystal on its own is deeply powerful, its energies can be magnified tenfold when connected with those of other stones in an intentional geometrical pattern, also known as a crystal grid. Crystal grids can be created for any purpose, using any combination of crystals. The below example will help you connect to the powerful unseen world.

You will need some combination of the following stones:

amethyst · azurite · calcite
clear quartz · kyanite
lapis lazuli · opal · shattuckite

You will need anywhere between 18 and 36 crystals in all. (It's useful, for geometrical and magical purposes, to work in multiples of three.) You will need one quartz point or selenite wand, as well.

There are crystal grid mats or printouts available online and in books, but it's much more creative (and therefore more powerful) to arrange your crystals by sight and feel. The goal is to create a balanced grid, so vary the dark and light colors of your crystals, rather than grouping them all together. If you have some that are wand-shaped rather than rounded, place them in opposition to each other. Aesthetics matter here.

When your grid is complete, take a moment to activate it. Starting from the outside and working your way in toward the center, use your quartz point or selenite wand to draw lines connecting each crystal, bringing them into alignment with each other. Focus your intentions as you do so, until you have reached the center stone.

For the purposes of this grid, it's a good idea to meditate over it, allowing the combined crystal energies to wash over you as you connect to the *something more* that exists in this world. After you're finished, you can leave the grid in place for as long as you like. Be sure to cleanse your crystals when you're ready to put them away.

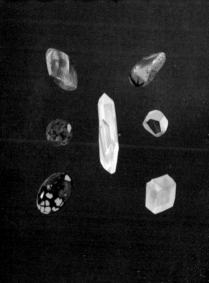

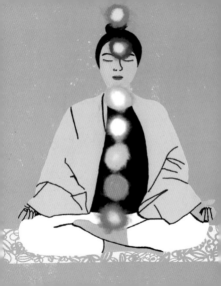

CRYSTALS
AND
CHAKRAS

THE CONNECTION BETWEEN
crystals and chakras stems from
a kind of logical-but-magical
correspondence. Like crystals,
chakras are manifestations of
frequency and energy. In some

ways, chakras are a lot less magical than they sound, for they are simply an ancient way of interpreting the endocrine system. A chakra is an energy center in the body and is generally visualized as a swirl found in a specific place along the spine (the word "chakra" is Sanskrit for "wheel"). There are seven of these swirls in all, starting at the base of the spine and reaching up to the crown of the head. They are connected to each other, and with the rest of the body, by "prana," the human life force—also known as energy meridians, nadis, qi, and many other names, including the peripheral nervous system. Qi Gong, Tai Chi, acupressure, acupuncture, EFT, reiki, and more all work with prana.

Each chakra has its own sound frequency as well as its

own light frequency (color). A chakra can be considered either "open," so that it is spinning and churning out energy, or "closed" or "blocked," so that it has stopped and your prana cannot move through it. In order for the body, mind, and spirit to be whole, each of these chakras needs to be open and balanced. A physical issue with a chakra can create an emotional or

mental issue, and an emotional
or mental issue that relates to a
chakra can produce a physical
response. The body is not
separate from your mind and
spirit; all three are intertwined,
and they influence each other
every moment of the day.

A blocked chakra can be
closed for a variety of reasons.
It can be something small, like
an unpleasant interaction at

work—which would likely create just a temporary blockage—or a severe emotional trauma—which would make it more difficult to reopen. If you experience a trauma, your chakra will respond to that experience by protecting itself—for example, if you lose a loved one, your closed heart chakra could cause you to develop asthma or bronchitis. A chakra can also be hyperactive and overpower the other chakras. This can mean that you are directing too much attention to the area of your life (from a mind, body, and spirit perspective) that is governed by that particular chakra.

In order for the body, mind, and spirit to be in harmony—so in order for you to live a harmonious life—your chakras need to be balanced. Each of them should have a free flow of energy moving both inward towards you and outwards toward the world. When your chakras are in balance, you feel at ease within your whole self, as you are giving and receiving freely with the world. Crystals can be a powerful tool in creating and maintaining balance between your chakras. In the next section, we'll explore the properties of the chakras to better understand how to utilize a crystal practice to foster alignment.

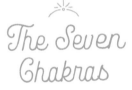

The Seven Chakras

Each of the chakras represents a certain aspect of the physical, emotional, and spiritual body in its own way. Each one is associated with a color, certain crystals, and a specific sound, which can be useful when chanting to open up the individual chakras.

MULADHARA The root chakra is located at the base of the spine, centered at the bladder and the colon. This is the most instinctual of all chakras—

our "fight or flight" response is located here. This chakra governs our connection with our ancestors, our past, and our literal roots in the earth. Everything else stems from here, as the other six chakras cannot be fully functional unless we have the support of the root chakra. When the root chakra is blocked, we might experience leg and foot pain, as well as problems with the lower digestive tract. When we are feeling worried about our basic survival needs—when that "fight or flight" response is in play—that might indicate a blocked root chakra as well. On the other hand, when we are being irresponsible about money, or about our personal safety, then that means the root chakra is overactive—and we are not as safe as we think we are. When the root

chakra is balanced we feel, and are, utterly fearless and safe. *Crystals:* obsidian, hematite, agate, bloodstone, bronzite, smoky quartz
Color: red or black *Sound:* Lam

SVADHISTHANA The

sacral chakra is just above the root chakra, where the ovaries and testes are located—and you guessed it, this chakra governs our creativity and sexuality. Pleasure and passion, both physical and spiritual, stem from this chakra. When it's blocked, we are literally blocked. Writer's block, artist's block, and an inability to be inspired, or even to feel pleasure, are all the result of a blocked sacral chakra. On the flip side, an overactive sacral chakra can provoke us to hedonistic or manic energies and behaviors. In either case, an imbalanced sacral chakra can cause physical problems like fertility issues, kidney trouble, or hip and lower back pain. But when the sacral chakra is balanced, we are more fertile in every way—we are sexually engaged and ripe with ideas and passions.

Crystals: sunstone, rutilated quartz, carnelian, garnet, ruby, citrine

Color: orange *Sound:* Vam-

MANIPURA The solar plexus chakra is located beneath the breastbone, near the adrenal glands and the endocrine system. Manipura is about personal power, our sense of self and our inner strength. This is where we find the source of our willpower, the drive that takes us from inertia to action. A blocked solar plexus means that the critical inner voice we all have is constantly shouting at us. We might fear rejection and relegate ourselves to the sidelines of our own lives, while those with an overactive solar plexus chakra might be overly dominating, overstressed, and may be in need of constant attention—someone who always demands the spotlight, whether it is positive or negative. Physical manifestations of imbalance include high blood pressure, chronic fatigue, and stomach ulcers. But a balanced solar plexus chakra gives us the confidence to make good choices in our lives. Someone with a balanced solar plexus chakra is assertive without being arrogant, and is in control without being afraid.

Crystals: tiger's eye, pyrite, yellow jasper, peridot, mookaite
Color: yellow *Sound:* Ram

ANAHATA The heart chakra is of course located at the heart, but also at the lungs. This central chakra is responsible for maintaining the balance between the other six. And how else to achieve that balance but with love, and with the breath and space to allow those we love to be who they are and love us in return? This love includes romantic love, self-love, friendship, kindness, compassion, and respect. This is how we recognize that we are not alone, that we are part of a community, of a partnership, of a family. When the heart chakra is blocked, we cannot feel that love—we cannot allow it into ourselves, and we cannot demonstrate it to others. And when it is overactive, we become needy and can have difficulty setting healthy bound-

aries. This can show up physically as asthma or even heart
disease, as well as shoulder and
upper back pain. But a balanced
heart chakra allows a life of love
and support, with all the joy and
space that brings.

Crystals: rose quartz, morganite,
malachite, emerald, rhodonite

Color: green or pink *Sound:* Yam

VISUDDHA The throat chakra is located near the thyroid gland. If the first three chakras are internal, and the heart is the balance, then the final three are about reaching outside of ourselves. The throat chakra is about speaking out, standing up for what we believe in, and showing up as our true selves with those around us. When we are afraid to speak out, or are presenting a version of ourselves to the world that isn't really true, then the throat chakra is blocked. On the other hand, if we are shouting at the world, and speaking without compassion or interest in others, then the throat chakra is overactive. This can manifest physically in a hyperactive or hypoactive thyroid, sore throat, neck pain, and mouth ulcers. A balanced throat chakra means that we not only speak the truth, but we can hear and accept it as well, as we live authentically in and with the world.

Crystals: aquamarine, turquoise, sodalite, blue lace agate

Color: light blue *Sound:* Ham

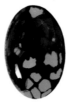

AJNA The third eye chakra is located near the pituitary gland. That third eye is a way of seeing things clearly. It's about observation and perception, but also wisdom—not just seeing, but seeing with truth and intuition. A blocked third eye cuts us off from the world around us, so that we look only within ourselves, until we become paranoid and depressed. But an overactive third eye can result in too much examination of the world outside, so that we imagine things about others that simply aren't true, and we become unfocused. Physical symptoms can include headaches, hearing loss, and blurred vision. But when the third eye chakra is balanced, we not only see what is happening around us, we comprehend it, feeling it deeply with compassion and understanding.

Crystals: lapis lazuli, azurite, fluorite, fuchsite, lepidolite, sapphire, labradorite, apophyllite

Color: indigo *Sound:* Ohm

SAHASRARA The crown chakra is located at the very top of the head, near the pineal gland and, of course, the brain. This chakra allows us to leave the self behind entirely, though of course it remains rooted in the other six chakras. Here we focus not just on what is outside the self, but what is *beyond* the self, beyond even the conception of self as it separates us from those

around us—and from the spiritual world. Sahasrara connects us
with all life, and with the magical
power of the spirit and the universe. When the crown chakra
is blocked we are isolated and
lonely, bitter and weighted by
the difficulties of life, and when
it is overactive we can become
arrogant, believing we know
more than we do, and holding
ourselves separate and above

those around us. Nightmares, migraines, and insomnia are the physical manifestations of this imbalance. But a balanced crown chakra allows us to find the best version of ourselves, that version that is tapped into the energy of all life.

Crystals: sugilite, opal, amethyst, kyanite, clear quartz, celestite, apophyllite

Color: purple *Sound:* Ahh

Crystal
Chakra
Ritual

Begin by allowing yourself time,
peace, and quiet. In order for
this ritual to be effective, you
need to be able to focus on it,
which means you need the space,

both physically and mentally, to do so. If you've got kids playing noisily in the background, that will distract you. If you've got your phone nearby, or if you're waiting on a phone call, that will be a distraction. If you're surrounded by unfolded laundry, unpaid bills, or any other work that has been left undone, that will be a distraction. That doesn't mean you have to go do all of

these things before performing
this ritual. Then it would never
get done, because our work in life
is never-ending! It just means
that you want to put yourself in
a place and frame of mind when
you won't be distracted by it. This
can be your bedroom, the floor, a
patch of grass, or anywhere else
you can lie flat, so long as it feels
calm. Allow yourself purity of
space. You can help this feeling

along by lighting candles, using an essential oil diffuser, burning sage or incense, playing gentle music—you know what works for you!

Gather at least one appropriate crystal for each chakra. It doesn't necessarily matter which one, and you can work with what you have handy, but if you have a specific intention for a certain chakra

and know that a particular crystal
will help with that intention,
then follow your intuition.
Cleanse and then program
each stone. Rather than using
a different cleansing method
for each, it's a good idea to treat
all of your crystals in the same
way for this ritual. Unless one
of them is particularly fragile,
it's a good idea to soak them all
together in a bowl of salt water,

as this will allow them to bond together and begin to work in harmony, even before the ritual begins. If you are using a more fragile crystal, wave a smudge wand over the stones as they are grouped together.

Program them individually. Hold one stone at a time, starting at the root chakra stones and working your way upward. If you are using more than one stone for a chakra, focus your intentions even more narrowly. So if, for instance, you are using obsidian and bloodstone for the root chakra, ask the obsidian to ground you, to hold you tethered to your ancestors, and ask the bloodstone to help you find your courage. Continue until each stone has received its intentions.

Once you've gathered, cleansed, and programmed your

stones, lie flat and ready them for placement: beginning at the root chakra, place your stone or stones at the base of your pubic bone, or on the ground just in front of it. Place your sacral chakra stone or stones just below your navel, and your solar plexus stones just below your ribcage. Place your heart chakra stones at your center, on your breastbone, and the throat chakra stone or stones in the hollow at the base of your throat. Place your third eye chakra stone or stones on your forehead just above and between your eyebrows, and place the crown chakra stone or stones off your head, just above it.

Lie flat, breathing deeply and evenly, as you allow the crystals to come into resonance with your chakras and with each other. When you've begun to feel their connection, move into chanting. If you don't feel anything, don't worry—that connection is there, and all you need to do is allow it. It's there even if you don't notice anything. Once you're relaxed, begin by focusing your attention on your root chakra. Feel the stones grow warm on your body, or if they are not touching you, feel their warmth and energy radiating toward you. Visualize the red and black colors of your root chakra, and watch them swirl as muladhara begins to allow and release a flow of energy. Breathe in deeply through your nose, and release the breath with a low, chanted "Laaaammmmmmm."

Once you feel an activation in your root chakra, which may show up as a softening, a warming, an energy, or even just a slight vibration, you can move on. Turning your attention to your sacral chakra, visualize an orange swirl beneath your crystal or crystals. You can even imagine the crystals floating on this vortex, or falling into it. Allow whatever comes to your mind. Breathe in deeply through your nose, and release the breath with a low, chanted "Vaaaammmmmm."

Continue in this manner up through each chakra, taking the time to focus your attention on each one in turn, seeing its color in your mind, feeling the weight and temperature of its crystal(s), and chanting its sound aloud. When you reach your crown chakra, focus your attention on the space *between* the top of your head and the crystal, for that is where your crown chakra is actually located. Feel the interplay between your energy and that of the crystal, and allow them both to enter the swirl of your crown chakra. Breathe in deeply through your nose, and exhale with a chanted "Ahhhhhhhhh."

As you move through each chakra, you may feel your body and your emotions responding more intensely to certain ones,

as you experience more heat, vibrations, or even emotional release. Allow it all.

When you've finished, visualize each chakra spinning together, united with the others. Allow their colors to spread and blend together, and the crystals to remain connected, until you feel yourself surrounded with a glow of white light. Breathe deeply and allow the energy to settle within you.

Don't get up right away.
Come back to your body, to
your present moment, but do
it slowly, allowing yourself to
make the journey with ease and
care. Remove your stones in the
reverse order that you placed
them. Take one last deep breath,
and release it before opening
your eyes.

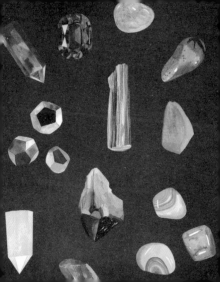